Complete Ulcerative Colitis Diet

A Complete Manual To Understanding Ulcerative Colitis With Easy & Quick Recipes to Permanent Control, Relieving Of Symptoms, Prevention And Improve your Well-Being.

Donna Johnson

Copyright 2024-

Donna Johnson

ISBN

Printed in the United States of America

Disclaimer

This publication is designed to provide competent and reliable information regarding the subject covered However, the views expressed in this publication are those of the author alone and should not be taken as expert instruction or professional advice The reader is responsible for his or her actions The author hereby disclaims any responsibility or liability whatsoever that is incurred from the use or application of the contents of this publication by the purchaser of the reader. The purchaser or reader is hereby responsible for his or her actions.

About The Book

Your go-to resource for controlling ulcerative colitis with diet is the "Complete Ulcerative Colitis Diet". Find time-tested techniques, nutrient-dense meals, and professional guidance to reduce symptoms and encourage recovery. Ascend to a revolutionary path towards healing and empower yourself to flourish beyond constraints. This is the starting point of your journey to a happy, fulfilled life.

About The Author

Donna Johnson is a skilled and enthusiastic dietician who is committed to advancing overall wellness and health. Motivated by her childhood and equipped with a Nutritional Sciences degree, she tackles nutrition with a combination of scientific precision and empathy. Donna is a natural at building relationships with people, creating individualized diet programs, and encouraging them to adopt better lives. She often offers her knowledge as a speaker and writer, encouraging others to put their health first. Donna is a trailblazer in the field of nutrition and health because of her contagious enthusiasm for life and unshakable dedication to serving others.

Table of Contents

Understanding Ulcerative Colitis and Diet Management

What is Ulcerative Colitis?

The chronic inflammatory bowel disease (IBD) known as ulcerative colitis (UC) is characterized by inflammation and ulcers in the lining of the colon and rectum. It is categorized as an inflammatory bowel illness, the same category that also includes Crohn's disease. While Crohn's disease may affect any portion of the digestive system, ulcerative colitis typically affects the colon and rectum. Despite these similarities, the two disorders are not the same.

Anatomy of the Colon and Rectum: Understanding the anatomy of the colon and rectum is crucial to understanding ulcerative colitis. The large intestine, or colon, is in charge of receiving water and electrolytes from food that has been digested and converting them into excrement. The ascending colon, transverse colon, descending colon, sigmoid colon, and rectum are its distinct portions. Before the anus, the rectum is the last segment of the large intestine where feces is held until it is eliminated.

Pathophysiology of Ulcerative Colitis: In those who are genetically susceptible to the condition, environmental stimuli are thought to provoke an aberrant immune response, which causes ulcerative colitis. Inadvertent immune system assaults on the colon and rectum lining cause tissue damage, inflammation, and ulcers. Although the precise etiology of this immunological dysregulation is not entirely known, a number of variables, including genetics, environmental triggers, and changes in the gut microbiota, are important.

Symptoms of Ulcerative Colitis:

The symptoms of ulcerative colitis can vary in severity and may include:

- Persistent diarrhea
- Abdominal pain and cramping
- Rectal bleeding
- Urgency to have a bowel movement
- Fatigue
- Weight loss
- Loss of appetite
- Fever

The symptoms often come and go, with periods of flare-ups and remission. Flare-ups can be debilitating and may require medical intervention to manage symptoms and prevent complications.

Diagnosis and Management: A study of the patient's medical history, a physical examination, laboratory testing, imaging investigations, and endoscopic procedures like sigmoidoscopy and colonoscopy are often used to diagnose ulcerative colitis. After a diagnosis, the goals of ulcerative colitis treatment are to enhance quality of life, reduce symptoms, avoid complications, and induce and sustain remission.

The Significance of Nutrition in the Management of Ulcerative Colitis: Although there is no cure for ulcerative colitis, nutrition is essential for symptom management, healing, and flare-up prevention. A diet that is well-balanced may promote gastrointestinal health, lower inflammation, provide vital nutrients, and enhance general wellbeing. Optimizing nutrient intake and reducing pain need knowing which foods to eat and which to avoid.

The principles of the ulcerative colitis diet, foods to include and avoid, meal planning techniques, and helpful hints for implementing dietary changes into your lifestyle to effectively manage ulcerative colitis and improve your quality of life will all be covered in detail in the sections that follow in this book.

Causes and Triggers of Ulcerative Colitis

The etiology of ulcerative colitis (UC) is diverse and complicated, with several contributing variables to both its development and aggravation.

1. Genetic Predisposition: There is compelling evidence that ulcerative colitis may have a hereditary component. People who have a family history of ulcerative colitis (UC) are more likely to have the illness. Certain genetic variants linked to the control of the immune system and inflammatory responses have been recognized as putative risk factors for ulcerative colitis.

2. Dysregulated immunological Response: A hallmark of ulcerative colitis is an aberrant immunological response. Environmental

factors may cause the immune system to launch an augmented reaction against the cells lining the colon and rectum in those with a hereditary susceptibility. The typical signs and symptoms of UC, including as diarrhea, stomach discomfort, and rectal bleeding, are brought on by this persistent inflammation.

3. Environmental variables: Environmental variables may cause ulcerative colitis to develop or worsen, even if genetics plays a major impact. The start and progression of ulcerative colitis (UC) may be influenced by environmental factors, including exposure to microbiological organisms, stress, smoking, and certain medicines, including nonsteroidal anti-inflammatory drugs. The precise processes by which these elements contribute to the pathophysiology of UC are still being studied, however.

4. Dysbiosis of the Gut Microbiota: The gastrointestinal tract's billions of bacteria, or gut microbiota, are essential for immune response regulation and intestinal homeostasis. Dysbiosis, or changes in the

makeup and activity of the gut microbiota, has been linked to ulcerative colitis patients. Intestinal inflammation and UC symptoms may be exacerbated by imbalances in the good-to-bad bacteria balance.

5. Dietary Triggers: Although a person's diet does not cause ulcerative colitis on its own, several dietary elements might make symptoms worse and produce flare-ups in those who are vulnerable. Typical dietary triggers include of: - Consuming large amounts of processed foods and refined sugars.

6. Dairy product consumption (particularly in those who are lactose intolerant)

   - Fried and fatty meals
   - Hot dishes
   - Caffeine and alcohol High-fiber meals in the event of a flare-up

7. Psychological Factors: Emotional and psychological stressors may affect how ulcerative colitis develops. Stress may affect

the immune system and the gut-brain axis, which can worsen symptoms and cause illness flare-ups. Using stress-reduction strategies like mindfulness, meditation, and relaxation exercises may enhance medical treatment and enhance the general well-being of people with ulcerative colitis.

Importance of Diet in Managing Ulcerative Colitis

Diet is a key component in the management of ulcerative colitis (UC), since it affects the degree of symptoms, the course of the illness, and general health. Although dietary changes by themselves may not be able to cure UC, they can greatly lessen symptoms, lower inflammation, and enhance the quality of life for those who suffer from this chronic illness.

1. Reducing Symptoms and Flare-Ups: For people with ulcerative colitis, a few foods and dietary practices may make symptoms worse and cause flare-ups. During active inflammation, common offenders include high-fat, high-spice, dairy, coffee, alcohol,

and high-fiber meals. People may lessen the intensity of their symptoms, ease their stomach pain, and restore regularity in their bowel movements by recognizing and removing certain food triggers.

2. Fostering Digestive Health: A diet high in antioxidants, prebiotic fibers, and nutrients that is well-balanced may help encourage the development of good gut flora and improve gut health. These microorganisms are essential for preserving the integrity of the intestinal barrier, regulating immunological responses, and lowering intestinal inflammation. Foods high in fruits, vegetables, whole grains, lean meats, omega-3 fatty acids, nuts, and seeds are especially good for the gut and may help reduce ulcerative colitis symptoms.

3. Improving vitamin Absorption: Because ulcerative colitis causes inflammation and damages the intestinal lining, it may hinder the absorption of nutrients and result in vitamin shortages. In people with UC, several nutrients such as iron, calcium, vitamin D,

vitamin B12, and folate may not be well absorbed or may be lost via diarrhea. In addition to preventing deficiencies and promoting general health and wellbeing, a diet high in nutrients that consists of a range of nutrient-rich foods may aid in the replacement of lost nutrients.

4. Promoting Healing and Remission: For those with ulcerative colitis, dietary therapies may aid in the healing process in addition to medical therapy. It has been shown that a few nutrients and bioactive substances contain anti-inflammatory qualities, which may aid in lowering intestinal inflammation. For instance, omega-3 fatty acids, which are included in walnuts, flaxseeds, and fatty fish, have been linked to better disease outcomes and reduced inflammation in UC patients.

5. Individualized Approach: It's critical to understand that dietary guidelines for ulcerative colitis should be customized to meet the specific requirements, dietary preferences, and tolerances of each person. What suits one individual may not be

appropriate for another. Maintaining a food journal, monitoring symptoms, and collaborating closely with a physician or registered dietitian may all aid in the identification of customized dietary plans that maximize symptom control and foster long-term remission.

6. Aspects of Psychology and Emotion: Adopting a nutritious diet may assist a person with ulcerative colitis's psychological and emotional well-being in addition to their physical health. The worry, despair, and stress that come with having a chronic disease may be lessened by feeling strong and in charge of one's food and way of life. Creating a network of support, engaging in mindfulness exercises, and getting professional therapy or attending support groups may all help to improve resilience and coping skills.

Common Symptoms and Challenges

The symptoms and difficulties associated with ulcerative colitis (UC) may have a serious negative effect on a person's quality of life. Comprehending these indications and obstacles is crucial for efficient handling and enhanced general welfare.

1. Constant Diarrhea: Constant diarrhea, often associated with urgency and frequent bowel motions, is one of the main symptoms of ulcerative colitis. The inflammation and ulceration of the colon and rectum cause diarrhea, which in turn causes a reduction in water absorption and an increase in the frequency of stools. Dietary adjustments, water, and sometimes medication are needed to manage diarrhea in order to minimize inflammation and restore bowel function.

2. Abdominal discomfort and Cramping: People who have ulcerative colitis often complain of stomach discomfort and cramping. Pain may range widely in intensity and location, from minor aches and pains to incapacitating cramping. When inflammation is elevated during flare-ups, abdominal discomfort often results. Painkillers, anti-inflammatory therapy, stress management methods, and

dietary changes are some methods of pain relief.

3. Rectal Bleeding: One upsetting sign of ulcerative colitis is rectal bleeding, which is often followed by blood in the stool. The colon's and the rectal lining's inflammation and ulcers are the causes of bleeding. While minor bleeding may stop on its own, significant bleeding has to be treated by a doctor in order to avoid problems including hemorrhage and anemia. Medication, dietary modifications, and in some situations, surgery, are possible forms of treatment.

4. Urgency to Have a Bowel Movement: People who have ulcerative colitis often feel the need to go to the bathroom urgently, particularly when they are having flare-ups. Urgency may cause anxiety and humiliation in addition to interfering with regular tasks. Identifying and avoiding trigger foods, keeping regular bowel habits, and making strategic use of restroom facilities to reduce pain and annoyance are some strategies to control urgency.

5. Weakness and Fatigue: Persistent ulcerative colitis symptoms and chronic inflammation might aggravate weakness and malaise. Anemia, dietary deficits, adverse drug reactions, and poor sleep quality may all make you feel more tired. Resolving the underlying reasons of exhaustion with dietary changes, supplements, stress reduction, and lifestyle improvements may help boost vitality and improve general health.

6. Effect on Emotion and Psychology: Having ulcerative colitis may have an adverse effect on one's emotional and psychological health. Treatment regimen management, adjusting to lifestyle changes, and coping with persistent illnesses may all contribute to stress, anxiety, depression, and social isolation. Enhancing coping abilities and fostering emotional resilience may be achieved via practicing mindfulness, getting professional counseling or therapy, creating a strong support system, and taking part in joyful activities.

7. Treatment Difficulties and Adherence: Medication, dietary adjustments, lifestyle modifications, and sometimes surgery are all often used in the treatment of ulcerative colitis. Treatment plan adherence might be difficult because of adverse drug reactions, dietary limitations, budgetary restraints, and psychological obstacles. Adherence may be facilitated and results can be optimized by establishing open contact with healthcare professionals, defining realistic objectives, and actively engaging in treatment choices.

Building a Healthy Diet Plan for Ulcerative Colitis

Principles of Ulcerative Colitis Diet

Understanding the subtleties of ulcerative colitis (UC) and implementing dietary practices that support symptom management, foster gut health, and improve general well-being are essential to creating a good diet plan. The following are the main ideas of a diet for ulcerative colitis:

Adopt a Low-Residue Diet: This diet calls for reducing the amount of high-fiber, difficult-to-digest meals. By lowering the frequency and amount of bowel movements, this lessens the inflammatory lining of the intestines' discomfort. A low-residue diet should consist of lean proteins, refined grains, soft fruits without seeds or skins, well-cooked veggies without skins, and dairy products in moderation.

Emphasize Foods That Are Easily Digested: Select meals that are simple to digest and mild on the digestive tract, especially when there are flare-ups or times of active inflammation. Choose soft, easily digested meals such cooked veggies, fish, eggs, chicken, white rice, oatmeal, and smooth nut butters. These foods should also be well-cooked and well-cooked.

Make Lean Proteins a Priority: To maintain muscular strength and mend tissue damage, include lean protein sources in your diet. Compared to fatty or highly processed meats, lean proteins like skinless chicken, fish, eggs, tofu, tempeh, and lentils are simpler to digest and less likely to aggravate UC symptoms.

Include Foods That Are Gut-Friendly: Select meals that encourage the development of good gut flora and gut health. Consume foods high in probiotics in moderation, such as yogurt, kefir, kombucha, sauerkraut, kimchi, and other fermented foods. These meals may lessen intestinal inflammation and aid in maintaining a balanced population of gut microbes.

Remain Hydrated: People with ulcerative colitis must always stay properly hydrated, particularly when they are experiencing diarrhea or are losing more fluids than usual. Throughout the day, sip on plenty of water to stay hydrated and replace any lost fluids. Carbonated and caffeinated drinks may aggravate the gastrointestinal system and worsen dehydration, therefore limit or stay away from them.

Watch out for FODMAPs: Certain forms of carbohydrates known as fermentable oligosaccharides, disaccharides, monosaccharides, and polyols (FODMAPS) may cause gastrointestinal symptoms including gas, bloating, and diarrhea in sensitive people, including those who have ulcerative colitis. To lessen pain in the digestive tract, try reducing your intake of high-FODMAP foods, which include certain fruits, vegetables, dairy products, cereals, and sweets.

Try Out Some Food Triggers: To track your food consumption and see how various foods impact your symptoms of UC, keep a food diary. To reduce the likelihood of symptom flare-ups, be aware of probable food triggers and think about removing or minimizing them from your diet. Caffeine, alcohol, dairy products, hot and fatty meals, and artificial additives are common triggers.

Take into Account Nutritional Supplements: To treat vitamin shortages or promote healing during flare-ups, people with ulcerative colitis may sometimes need to take nutritional supplements. Consult a qualified dietitian or your healthcare professional about the best supplement choices for you given your unique requirements and current nutritional state.

Foods to Include for Managing Symptoms

A well-thought-out diet is essential for ulcerative colitis (UC) sufferers to manage their symptoms and maintain general health. Although dietary preferences and tolerances differ from person to person, there are several foods that are typically well-tolerated and may help reduce the symptoms of ulcerative colitis.

Low-Residue Foods: Incorporating low-residue foods into your diet can help reduce the frequency and severity of bowel movements, minimize abdominal discomfort, and alleviate symptoms of ulcerative colitis during flare-ups. Low-residue foods are low in fiber and are less likely to irritate the digestive tract. Examples include:

- Refined grains such as white rice, white bread, and pasta
- Cooked fruits and vegetables without skins or seeds (e.g., peeled apples, peeled and cooked carrots)
- Tender and well-cooked meats, poultry, and fish
- Eggs
- Dairy alternatives such as lactose-free milk and yogurt

Lean Proteins: Including lean proteins in your diet provides essential amino acids necessary for tissue repair, muscle maintenance, and overall health. Opt for lean sources of protein that are easy to digest and gentle on the stomach. Examples include:

- Skinless poultry (e.g., chicken, turkey)
- Fish (e.g., salmon, trout, tilapia)
- Lean cuts of beef and pork
- Eggs

- Tofu and tempeh

Omega-3 Fatty Acids: Omega-3 fatty acids possess anti-inflammatory properties and may help reduce inflammation in the gut, thereby alleviating symptoms of ulcerative colitis. Incorporate foods rich in omega-3 fatty acids into your diet to support gut health and promote overall well-being. Sources of omega-3 fatty acids include:

- Fatty fish such as salmon, mackerel, sardines, and trout
- Flaxseeds and flaxseed oil
- Chia seeds
- Walnuts

Probiotic-Rich Foods: Probiotics are beneficial bacteria that support digestive health, promote gut microbiota balance, and strengthen the immune system. Consuming probiotic-rich foods may help alleviate symptoms of ulcerative colitis and improve gastrointestinal function. Consider adding the following probiotic-rich foods to your diet:

- Yogurt with live active cultures
- Kefir

- Fermented vegetables such as sauerkraut, kimchi, and pickles (choose varieties without added sugars or high salt content)
- Kombucha

Hydration: People with ulcerative colitis must drink enough of water, particularly when they are experiencing flare-ups that include diarrhea and fluid loss. Drink a lot of water over the day to keep your electrolyte balance stable and avoid dehydration. To keep hydrated and promote gastrointestinal health, choose electrolyte-rich liquids, diluted fruit juices, herbal teas, and water.

Foods to Avoid or Limit

While certain foods may help people with ulcerative colitis (UC) manage their symptoms and maintain gut health, others might make symptoms worse, cause flare-ups, or cause pain in the digestive tract. Knowing which foods to restrict or avoid may help reduce the intensity of symptoms and improve UC treatment.

High-Fiber Foods: Although meals high in fiber are usually good for digestive health, people with UC may find it difficult to tolerate them, particularly during flare-ups. Foods high in fiber may cause diarrhea, bloating, and cramping in the abdomen by increasing the size and frequency of stools. Eat less of or steer clear of the following high-fiber foods:

- Whole grains such as whole wheat, whole grain bread, and brown rice
- Bran cereals and oatmeal
- Nuts and seeds
- Legumes such as beans, lentils, and chickpeas
- Raw fruits and vegetables with skins or seeds

Dairy Products: Dairy products include lactose, a sugar that may be hard for people with UC to digest, especially if they have a lactose intolerance or have flare-ups. Consuming dairy products may make symptoms like diarrhea, bloating, stomach discomfort, and gas worse. Limit or stay away from the following dairy products:

- Cheese
- Milk
- Smoothies

- Ice cream

Spicy and Irritating meals: People with UC may experience gastrointestinal distress and inflammation as a result of eating spicy or highly flavorful or irritating meals. These meals may make symptoms like diarrhea, cramps, and stomach discomfort worse. Eat less of or stay away from the following hot and irritating foods:

- Hot sauces and spicy peppers
- Cayenne pepper and chili powder - Vinegar and acidic foods (such as tomatoes and citrus fruits)
- Beverages with caffeine and alcohol

Fried and Fatty meals: Fried and fatty meals include a lot of saturated and trans fats, which the digestive system may find difficult to handle and which may make ulcerative colitis symptoms worse. These foods may exacerbate stomach pain, lengthen the time it takes for the intestine to empty, and cause diarrhea. Reduce your intake of the following high-fat, fried foods:

- Fried meals, including fried chicken, French fries, and potato chips
- Fatty and greasy meats
- Processed meals that are rich in trans and saturated fats, such as cookies, pastries, and processed meats

Artificial Sweeteners and Food Additives: For people who have ulcerative colitis, artificial sweeteners and food additives may make symptoms worse and cause pain in the digestive tract. These chemicals have the potential to upset the equilibrium of gut bacteria and cause intestinal inflammation. Avoid or use in moderation the following artificial additives and sweeteners:

- Aspartame (found in sugar-free and diet beverages)
- Sucralose (found in drinks and chewing gum without added sugar).
- Saccharin, which is present in diet meals and drinks.
- Artificial preservatives and colorings for food

Importance of Hydration

A vital component of treating ulcerative colitis (UC) and preserving general health and wellbeing is staying hydrated. For healthy digestion, nutritional absorption, stool regularity, and general gastrointestinal function, one must drink enough water. Diarrhea is a common cause of excessive fluid loss in people with UC, which, if left untreated, may result in electrolyte imbalances and dehydration.

UC's Effect Signs of Dehydration: Dehydration may occur during ulcerative colitis flare-ups due to increased fluid loss and frequent diarrhea. When the body loses more fluid than it takes in, it becomes dehydrated and imbalances in electrolytes like sodium, potassium, and chloride happen. Dehydration may make UC symptoms worse, such as weakness, weariness, lightheadedness, and reduced urine production.

The Significance of Electrolyte Balance: Electrolytes are essential for preserving the body's pH balance, muscular contraction, neuron function, and fluid equilibrium. Particularly sodium, potassium, and chloride electrolyte deficits may result from diarrhea related to ulcerative colitis. It is essential to ensure proper hydration and electrolyte balance to avoid consequences such myofascial spasms, arrhythmias, and compromised cognitive abilities.

Hydration Techniques for UC Patients: In order to preserve electrolyte balance and be well hydrated, people with ulcerative colitis should follow these hydration guidelines:

- Drink Plenty of Fluids: If you're having diarrhea or losing a lot of fluid, try to drink at least 8 to 10 cups (64 to 80 ounces) of fluid per day. While water is the ideal beverage for hydration, other liquids may also help you stay hydrated, including clear broths, diluted fruit juices, herbal teas, and sports drinks with plenty of electrolytes.

- Pay Attention to Urine Color: Urine color might provide information about hydration levels. While dark yellow or amber-colored urine may suggest dehydration and the need to increase fluid intake, pale yellow pee indicates appropriate hydration.

- Replace Electrolytes: To replace electrolytes lost due to diarrhea, think about ingesting electrolyte-rich drinks or oral rehydration treatments in addition to water. Sports beverages, electrolyte-containing rehydration packs, and coconut water may all assist in restoring electrolyte balance and preventing dehydration.

- Restrict Alcohol and Caffeine: Both substances have diuretic properties that might raise urine output and exacerbate dehydration. Restrict your use of alcoholic and caffeinated drinks, such as soda, coffee, and tea, particularly while your UC is flare-up.

- Include Hydrating Foods: Incorporate foods rich in water content, such as fruits (watermelon, oranges, strawberries), vegetables (cucumber, celery, lettuce), and soups, into your diet in addition to fluids.

- Track Weight Loss: Keep a constant eye on your weight since a noticeable drop in weight may be an indication of electrolyte imbalances and dehydration.

Strategies for Meal Timing and Portion Control

Timing meals well and controlling portion sizes are crucial for controlling ulcerative colitis (UC) and reducing symptoms including diarrhea, bloating, and pain in the abdomen. In people with UC, using deliberate meal timing and quantity management measures may assist promote digestion, enhance nutritional absorption, and regulate bowel movements.

Regular Meal pattern: For people with ulcerative colitis, maintaining a regular meal pattern may help control bowel movements and improve gastrointestinal health. Eat meals and snacks at regular intervals throughout the day to promote healthy digestion and reduce energy swings. Timing meals consistently may also aid in retraining the body's internal clock and encourage more regular bowel movements.

Small, Frequent Meals: Think about having smaller, more frequent meals and snacks throughout the day as an alternative to big, hefty ones. Smaller meals lower the risk of gastrointestinal distress and bloating because they are simpler to digest and less likely to overburden the digestive system. To provide your body a consistent supply of energy and nutrients without overburdening your digestive system, aim for four to six smaller meals spread out evenly throughout the day.

Mindful Eating: To improve awareness of fullness and hunger signals, avoid overindulging, and encourage healthy digestion, engage in mindful eating practices. Prior to eating, pause to evaluate your degree of hunger and pay attention to your body's signals of fullness and appetite. Chew food well, eat slowly, and enjoy every meal to aid in digestion and to help you feel full and satisfied.

Portion Control: Watch how much you consume and try not to overindulge, particularly when it comes to items that can make your ulcerative colitis symptoms worse. To estimate proper serving sizes, use visual clues like portion control plates, measuring cups, and hand portions. In order to reduce pain, pay attention to portion sizes of meals heavy in fiber, fat, or spice, as well as other items that may provoke UC symptoms.

Balanced Meals: To promote general health and wellbeing, concentrate on preparing balanced meals that include a range of nutrient-dense foods from all dietary categories. For optimal nutrition delivery, satiety, and blood sugar regulation, include lean proteins, complex carbs, healthy fats, and fiber-rich fruits and vegetables into your meals. Try out several meal combos and food pairings to see what suits your own requirements and tastes the best.

Hydration with Meals: To aid in digestion and avoid dehydration, particularly during ulcerative colitis flare-ups marked by increased fluid loss, stay hydrated by consuming fluids with meals. To stay as hydrated as possible during the day, choose electrolyte-rich drinks, diluted fruit juices, herbal teas, or water to go with meals and snacks.

Recipes and Meal Plans

Breakfast Recipes for Ulcerative Colitis Diet

Banana Oat Pancakes	Ingredients: Rolled oats, ripe banana, egg, cinnamon.
	Instructions: Blend oats into flour, mix with mashed banana, egg, and cinnamon. Cook on a non-stick pan until golden brown.
	Preparation time: 15 minutes.
Scrambled Tofu Breakfast Bowl	Ingredients: Firm tofu, spinach, cherry tomatoes, olive oil, turmeric.
	Instructions: Sauté spinach, tomatoes, and crumbled tofu with turmeric until heated through.
	Preparation time: 15 minutes.
Quinoa Breakfast Porridge	Ingredients: Quinoa, almond milk, honey, sliced almonds.
	Instructions: Cook quinoa in almond milk until fluffy, sweeten with honey, and top with sliced almonds.
	Preparation time: 20 minutes.

Greek Yogurt Parfait	Ingredients: Greek yogurt, granola, honey, mixed berries.
	Instructions: Layer yogurt, granola, and berries in a glass, drizzle with honey.
	Preparation time: 5 minutes.
Rice Cake with Almond Butter and Sliced Banana	Ingredients: Rice cake, almond butter, banana.
	Instructions: Spread almond butter on rice cake, top with sliced banana.
	Preparation time: 5 minutes.
Egg White Omelette with Spinach and Mushrooms	Ingredients: Egg whites, baby spinach, mushrooms, olive oil.
	Instructions: Sauté spinach and mushrooms, add egg whites, cook until set.
	Preparation time: 10 minutes.
Chia Seed Pudding with Berries	Ingredients: Chia seeds, almond milk, vanilla extract, maple syrup, mixed berries.
	Instructions: Mix chia seeds with almond milk, vanilla, and maple syrup. Refrigerate overnight, serve with mixed berries.

	Preparation time: 5 minutes (+overnight refrigeration).
Cottage Cheese and Pineapple Bowl	Ingredients: Cottage cheese, fresh pineapple chunks.
	Instructions: Serve cottage cheese topped with pineapple chunks.
	Preparation time: 5 minutes.
Brown Rice Porridge with Cinnamon and Raisins	Ingredients: Brown rice, almond milk, cinnamon, raisins.
	Instructions: Cook brown rice in almond milk until creamy, stir in cinnamon and raisins.
	Preparation time: 25 minutes.
Spinach and Banana Smoothie	Ingredients: Baby spinach, ripe banana, almond milk.
	Instructions: Blend spinach, banana, and almond milk until smooth.
	Preparation time: 5 minutes.
Avocado Toast	Ingredients: Ripe avocado, whole grain bread, lemon juice.
	Instructions: Mash avocado with lemon juice, spread on toast.
	Preparation time: 5 minutes.

Buckwheat Pancakes with Blueberries	Ingredients: Buckwheat flour, almond milk, baking powder, blueberries.
	Instructions: Mix batter, fold in blueberries, cook until golden brown.
	Preparation time: 20 minutes.
Papaya Boat with Yogurt and Granola	Ingredients: Papaya, Greek yogurt, granola.
	Instructions: Fill papaya halves with yogurt, sprinkle with granola.
	Preparation time: 10 minutes.
Apple Slices with Almond Butter	Ingredients: Apple, almond butter.
	Instructions: Slice apple, serve with almond butter.
	Preparation time: 5 minutes.
Turkey and Lettuce Wrap	Ingredients: Sliced turkey breast, lettuce leaves.
	Instructions: Wrap turkey slices in lettuce leaves.
	Preparation time: 10 minutes.
	Ingredients: Millet, almond milk, cinnamon, raisins.

Millet Porridge with Cinnamon and Raisins	Instructions: Cook millet in almond milk until tender, stir in cinnamon and raisins.
	Preparation time: 25 minutes.
Soft Boiled Eggs with Whole Grain Toast Soldiers	Ingredients: Eggs, whole grain bread.
	Instructions: Soft boil eggs, serve with toast soldiers.
	Preparation time: 10 minutes.
Spinach and Mushroom Frittata	Ingredients: Eggs, baby spinach, mushrooms, onion.
	Instructions: Sauté vegetables, add beaten eggs, bake until set.
	Preparation time: 20 minutes.
Apple Cinnamon Overnight Oats	Ingredients: Rolled oats, almond milk, apple slices, cinnamon.
	Instructions: Mix oats, milk, apple, and cinnamon. Refrigerate overnight.
	Preparation time: 5 minutes (+overnight refrigeration).
Sweet Potato Hash with Bell Peppers	Ingredients: Sweet potato, bell peppers, olive oil.
	Instructions: Sauté sweet potato and peppers until tender.

	Preparation time: 20 minutes.
Rice Cakes with Smoked Salmon and Dill	Ingredients: Rice cakes, smoked salmon, fresh dill.
	Instructions: Top rice cakes with salmon and dill.
	Preparation time: 10 minutes.
Gluten-Free Blueberry Muffins	Ingredients: Almond flour, blueberries, honey.
	Instructions: Mix ingredients, bake until golden.
	Preparation time: 25 minutes.
Peanut Butter and Banana Smoothie	Ingredients: Peanut butter, ripe banana, almond milk.
	Instructions: Blend ingredients until smooth.
	Preparation time: 5 minutes.
Cantaloupe with Cottage Cheese	Ingredients: Cantaloupe, cottage cheese.
	Instructions: Serve cottage cheese in cantaloupe halves.
	Preparation time: 5 minutes.
Vegetable Frittata	Ingredients: Eggs, zucchini, cherry tomatoes, onion.
	Instructions: Sauté vegetables, add beaten eggs, bake until set.

	Preparation time: 20 minutes.
Almond Flour Pancakes	Ingredients: Almond flour, eggs, baking powder.
	Instructions: Mix batter, cook until golden.
	Preparation time: 15 minutes.
Fruit Salad with Honey-Lime Dressing	Ingredients: Assorted fruits, lime juice, honey.
	Instructions: Toss fruits with lime juice and honey.
	Preparation time: 10 minutes.
Rice Porridge with Ginger and Turmeric	Ingredients: Rice, ginger, turmeric.
	Instructions: Cook rice with ginger and turmeric until soft.
	Preparation time: 30 minutes.
Tomato and Basil Omelette	Ingredients: Eggs, cherry tomatoes, fresh basil.
	Instructions: Cook eggs with tomatoes and basil.
	Preparation time: 15 minutes.
Cucumber and Avocado Smoothie	Ingredients: Cucumber, avocado, spinach, almond milk.
	Instructions: Blend ingredients until smooth.

	Preparation time: 5 minutes.
Rice Cake with Cottage Cheese and Sliced Strawberries	Ingredients: Rice cake, cottage cheese, strawberries.
	Instructions: Spread cottage cheese on rice cake, top with strawberries.
	Preparation time: 5 minutes.
Turkey Sausage Patties	Ingredients: Ground turkey, sage, thyme.
	Instructions: Mix ingredients, shape into patties, cook until browned.
	Preparation time: 20 minutes.
Mango and Coconut Chia Pudding	Ingredients: Chia seeds, mango, coconut milk.
	Instructions: Mix chia seeds with coconut milk, layer with mango. Refrigerate overnight.
	Preparation time: 5 minutes (+overnight refrigeration).
Almond Butter Toast with Sliced Kiwi	Ingredients: Whole grain toast, almond butter, kiwi.
	Instructions: Spread almond butter on toast, top with kiwi slices.

	Preparation time: 5 minutes.
Oat Bran Porridge with Raspberries	Ingredients: Oat bran, almond milk, raspberries.
	Instructions: Cook oat bran in almond milk, top with raspberries.
	Preparation time: 15 minutes.
Egg and Spinach Breakfast Wrap	Ingredients: Whole grain wrap, eggs, baby spinach.
	Instructions: Cook eggs, spinach, wrap in tortilla.
	Preparation time: 10 minutes.
Baked Apple with Cinnamon and Walnuts	Ingredients: Apple, cinnamon, walnuts.
	Instructions: Core apple, sprinkle with cinnamon and walnuts, bake until tender.
	Preparation time: 30 minutes.
Greek Yogurt with Muesli and Banana Slices	Ingredients: Greek yogurt, muesli, banana.
	Instructions: Layer yogurt, muesli, banana slices.
	Preparation time: 5 minutes.
Brown Rice Cake with Almond	Ingredients: Brown rice cake, almond butter, pear.

Butter and Sliced Pear	Instructions: Spread almond butter on rice cake, top with pear slices.
	Preparation time: 5 minutes.
Tofu Scramble Breakfast Burrito	Ingredients: Firm tofu, bell peppers, onions, whole grain tortilla.
	Instructions: Sauté tofu, peppers, onions, fill tortilla.
	Preparation time: 20 minutes.
Poached Eggs with Steamed Asparagus	Ingredients: Eggs, asparagus.
	Instructions: Poach eggs, steam asparagus until tender.
	Preparation time: 15 minutes.
Rice Porridge with Miso and Green Onions	Ingredients: Rice, miso paste, green onions.
	Instructions: Cook rice with miso, garnish with green onions.
	Preparation time: 30 minutes.
Pumpkin Spice Smoothie	Ingredients: Pumpkin puree, banana, almond milk, cinnamon.
	Instructions: Blend ingredients until smooth.
	Preparation time: 5 minutes.

Chickpea Flour Pancakes	Ingredients: Chickpea flour, water, baking powder.
	Instructions: Mix batter, cook until golden.
	Preparation time: 15 minutes.
Fruit and Nut Breakfast Couscous	Ingredients: Whole wheat couscous, mixed dried fruits, almonds.
	Instructions: Cook couscous, stir in fruits and nuts.
	Preparation time: 15 minutes.
Cottage Cheese Pancakes	Ingredients: Cottage cheese, eggs, oat flour.
	Instructions: Mix ingredients, cook until golden.
	Preparation time: 20 minutes.
Kiwi and Orange Smoothie	Ingredients: Kiwi, orange, spinach, almond milk.
	Instructions: Blend ingredients until smooth.
	Preparation time: 5 minutes.
Vegetable and Turkey Bacon Egg Muffins	Ingredients: Eggs, turkey bacon, bell peppers, spinach.
	Instructions: Mix ingredients, bake in muffin tin until set.

	Preparation time: 25 minutes.

Lunch and Dinner Recipes for Ulcerative Colitis Diet

Grilled Chicken Salad	Ingredients: Grilled chicken breast, mixed greens, cucumber, cherry tomatoes, olive oil, lemon juice.
	Instructions: Toss ingredients together, drizzle with olive oil and lemon juice.
	Preparation time: 20 minutes.
Salmon with Steamed Asparagus	Ingredients: Salmon fillet, asparagus, olive oil, lemon slices.
	Instructions: Season salmon, steam asparagus, serve with lemon slices.
	Preparation time: 15 minutes.
Turkey and Quinoa Stuffed Peppers	Ingredients: Bell peppers, ground turkey, cooked quinoa, tomato sauce, Italian seasoning.
	Instructions: Stuff peppers with turkey-quinoa mixture, bake until tender.
	Preparation time: 30 minutes.

Vegetable Stir-Fry	Ingredients: Assorted vegetables (bell peppers, broccoli, carrots), tofu or chicken strips, soy sauce, ginger, garlic.
	Instructions: Stir-fry vegetables and protein in soy sauce, ginger, and garlic.
	Preparation time: 25 minutes.
Baked Cod with Lemon and Herbs	Ingredients: Cod fillet, lemon juice, fresh herbs (such as parsley or dill), olive oil.
	Instructions: Season cod with lemon juice, herbs, and olive oil, bake until flaky.
	Preparation time: 20 minutes.
Quinoa and Vegetable Salad	Ingredients: Cooked quinoa, mixed vegetables (cucumber, tomatoes, bell peppers), lemon vinaigrette.
	Instructions: Toss quinoa and vegetables with lemon vinaigrette.
	Preparation time: 15 minutes.
Shrimp and Zucchini Noodles	Ingredients: Shrimp, zucchini, garlic, olive oil, cherry tomatoes.

	Instructions: Sauté shrimp and zucchini noodles with garlic and cherry tomatoes.
	Preparation time: 20 minutes.
Turkey Meatball Soup	Ingredients: Ground turkey, carrots, celery, low-sodium chicken broth, thyme, parsley.
	Instructions: Form turkey meatballs, simmer with vegetables and broth.
	Preparation time: 35 minutes.
Roasted Vegetable Quinoa Bowl	Ingredients: Roasted vegetables (sweet potatoes, Brussels sprouts, cauliflower), cooked quinoa, tahini dressing.
	Instructions: Arrange vegetables and quinoa in a bowl, drizzle with tahini dressing.
	Preparation time: 30 minutes.
Grilled Lemon Herb Chicken	Ingredients: Chicken breasts, lemon zest, garlic, rosemary, olive oil.
	Instructions: Marinate chicken in lemon zest, garlic, rosemary, grill until cooked through.

	Preparation time: 25 minutes.
Salmon and Avocado Salad	Ingredients: Grilled salmon, mixed greens, avocado, cucumber, lemon vinaigrette.
	Instructions: Combine ingredients, toss with lemon vinaigrette.
	Preparation time: 20 minutes.
Vegetable and Lentil Soup	Ingredients: Lentils, carrots, celery, onion, vegetable broth, cumin, coriander.
	Instructions: Simmer lentils and vegetables in broth with spices until tender.
	Preparation time: 40 minutes.
Eggplant and Tomato Bake	Ingredients: Eggplant, tomatoes, garlic, basil, olive oil.
	Instructions: Layer sliced eggplant and tomatoes, drizzle with olive oil, bake until tender.
	Preparation time: 30 minutes.
Turkey and Vegetable Skewers	Ingredients: Turkey breast, bell peppers, zucchini, cherry tomatoes, olive oil, Italian seasoning.

	Instructions: Skewer turkey and vegetables, grill until cooked.
	Preparation time: 25 minutes.
Quinoa and Black Bean Salad	Ingredients: Cooked quinoa, black beans, corn, red onion, cilantro, lime juice.
	Instructions: Mix ingredients, toss with lime juice.
	Preparation time: 20 minutes.
Baked Chicken Thighs with Roasted Vegetables	Ingredients: Chicken thighs, potatoes, carrots, onions, garlic, thyme, olive oil.
	Instructions: Season chicken and vegetables, roast until golden.
	Preparation time: 40 minutes.
Tuna Salad Lettuce Wraps	Ingredients: Canned tuna, celery, red onion, Greek yogurt, Dijon mustard, lettuce leaves.
	Instructions: Mix tuna, celery, onion, yogurt, and mustard, spoon into lettuce leaves.
	Preparation time: 15 minutes.
Miso-Glazed Salmon	Ingredients: Salmon fillet, miso paste, soy sauce, honey, ginger.

	Instructions: Mix miso, soy sauce, honey, and ginger, glaze salmon, bake until cooked through.
	Preparation time: 25 minutes.
Turkey and Vegetable Stir-Fry	Ingredients: Ground turkey, mixed vegetables (snap peas, bell peppers, carrots), soy sauce, garlic, ginger.
	Instructions: Sauté turkey and vegetables with soy sauce, garlic, and ginger.
	Preparation time: 20 minutes.
Roasted Butternut Squash Soup	Ingredients: Butternut squash, onion, garlic, vegetable broth, coconut milk, nutmeg.
	Instructions: Roast squash and onion, blend with broth, coconut milk, and nutmeg.
	Preparation time: 45 minutes.
Grilled Lemon Garlic Shrimp	Ingredients: Shrimp, garlic, lemon juice, olive oil, parsley.
	Instructions: Marinate shrimp in garlic, lemon juice, and oil, grill until cooked.
	Preparation time: 15 minutes.

Stuffed Portobello Mushrooms	Ingredients: Portobello mushrooms, quinoa, spinach, feta cheese, cherry tomatoes.
	Instructions: Fill mushrooms with quinoa, spinach, feta, and tomatoes, bake until tender.
	Preparation time: 30 minutes.
Chicken and Vegetable Curry	Ingredients: Chicken breast, cauliflower, bell peppers, onion, curry paste, coconut milk.
	Instructions: Sauté chicken and vegetables, add curry paste and coconut milk, simmer until tender.
	Preparation time: 35 minutes.
Salmon Caesar Salad	Ingredients: Grilled salmon, romaine lettuce, cherry tomatoes, Caesar dressing, Parmesan cheese.
	Instructions: Combine ingredients, toss with Caesar dressing, top with Parmesan.
	Preparation time: 20 minutes.
Turkey and Brown Rice	Ingredients: Ground turkey, brown rice, bell peppers, tomato sauce, Italian seasoning.

Stuffed Bell Peppers	Instructions: Fill peppers with turkey-rice mixture, bake until peppers are soft.
	Preparation time: 40 minutes.
Lemon Herb Roasted Chicken	Ingredients: Chicken thighs or breasts, lemon zest, thyme, rosemary, olive oil.
	Instructions: Marinate chicken in lemon zest, herbs, and oil, roast until golden.
	Preparation time: 30 minutes.
Eggplant and Chickpea Tagine	Ingredients: Eggplant, chickpeas, tomatoes, onion, garlic, cumin, coriander, cinnamon.
	Instructions: Simmer ingredients with spices until tender.
	Preparation time: 40 minutes.
Tofu and Vegetable Lettuce Wraps	Ingredients: Firm tofu, mushrooms, water chestnuts, soy sauce, ginger, lettuce leaves.
	Instructions: Sauté tofu and vegetables with soy sauce and ginger, spoon into lettuce leaves.
	Preparation time: 25 minutes.

Salmon and Vegetable Foil Packets	Ingredients: Salmon fillets, zucchini, squash, bell peppers, lemon slices, dill.
	Instructions: Place salmon and vegetables on foil, season with lemon and dill, bake until cooked.
	Preparation time: 25 minutes.
Quinoa and Chickpea Pilaf	Ingredients: Cooked quinoa, chickpeas, spinach, garlic, lemon juice, olive oil.
	Instructions: Sauté chickpeas, spinach, and garlic, mix with quinoa, dress with lemon juice and oil.
	Preparation time: 25 minutes.
Chicken and Vegetable Kabobs	Ingredients: Chicken breast, bell peppers, onions, cherry tomatoes, olive oil, Italian seasoning.
	Instructions: Skewer chicken and vegetables, grill until chicken is cooked through.
	Preparation time: 30 minutes.

Turkey and Brown Rice Soup	Ingredients: Ground turkey, carrots, celery, onion, brown rice, chicken broth, thyme.
	Instructions: Simmer turkey, vegetables, rice, and broth with thyme until flavors meld.
	Preparation time: 40 minutes.
Vegetable and Tofu Stir-Fry	Ingredients: Tofu, broccoli, snap peas, carrots, soy sauce, garlic, ginger.
	Instructions: Sauté tofu and vegetables with soy sauce, garlic, and ginger.
	Preparation time: 25 minutes.
Baked Halibut with Herbed Butter	Ingredients: Halibut fillets, butter, parsley, lemon zest, garlic.
	Instructions: Mix butter with herbs and zest, spread on halibut, bake until flaky.
	Preparation time: 25 minutes.
Mushroom and Spinach Risotto	Ingredients: Arborio rice, mushrooms, spinach, onion, garlic, vegetable broth, Parmesan cheese.

	Instructions: Sauté mushrooms, onion, and garlic, stir in rice and broth, cook until creamy, stir in spinach and cheese.
	Preparation time: 40 minutes.
Turkey and Sweet Potato Skillet	Ingredients: Ground turkey, sweet potatoes, bell peppers, onion, cumin, paprika.
	Instructions: Sauté turkey and vegetables with spices until cooked through.
	Preparation time: 30 minutes.
Baked Chicken with Roasted Vegetables	Ingredients: Chicken thighs or breasts, potatoes, carrots, onion, garlic, thyme, olive oil.
	Instructions: Season chicken and vegetables, roast until golden.
	Preparation time: 40 minutes.
Lemon Garlic Shrimp Pasta	Ingredients: Shrimp, whole wheat pasta, garlic, lemon juice, parsley, olive oil.
	Instructions: Cook pasta, sauté shrimp with garlic, lemon, and oil, toss with pasta and parsley.
	Preparation time: 30 minutes.

Vegetable and Lentil Stew	Ingredients: Lentils, carrots, celery, onion, garlic, vegetable broth, thyme, bay leaf.
	Instructions: Simmer lentils and vegetables with broth and spices until tender.
	Preparation time: 45 minutes.
Salmon Cakes with Greek Yogurt Dill Sauce	Ingredients: Canned salmon, breadcrumbs, egg, Greek yogurt, dill, lemon juice.
	Instructions: Mix salmon, breadcrumbs, and egg, form into cakes, pan-fry until golden, serve with yogurt sauce.
	Preparation time: 30 minutes.
Turkey and Vegetable Curry	Ingredients: Ground turkey, cauliflower, bell peppers, onion, garlic, curry powder, coconut milk.
	Instructions: Sauté turkey and vegetables with curry powder, add coconut milk, simmer until flavors meld.
	Preparation time: 35 minutes.

Eggplant and Tomato Pasta	Ingredients: Eggplant, tomatoes, garlic, onion, whole wheat pasta, basil, olive oil.
	Instructions: Sauté eggplant, tomatoes, garlic, and onion, toss with cooked pasta, basil, and oil.
	Preparation time: 35 minutes.
Chicken and Vegetable Skillet	Ingredients: Chicken breast, bell peppers, zucchini, cherry tomatoes, garlic, Italian seasoning.
	Instructions: Sauté chicken and vegetables with garlic and seasoning until cooked through.
	Preparation time: 25 minutes.
Quinoa and Black Bean Stuffed Bell Peppers	Ingredients: Cooked quinoa, black beans, corn, tomatoes, chili powder, cumin, bell peppers.
	Instructions: Mix quinoa, beans, corn, tomatoes, and spices, stuff into peppers, bake until tender.
	Preparation time: 40 minutes.
Tofu and Vegetable Curry	Ingredients: Firm tofu, cauliflower, peas, carrots, onion, curry paste, coconut milk.

	Instructions: Sauté tofu and vegetables with curry paste, add coconut milk, simmer until flavors meld.
	Preparation time: 35 minutes.
Salmon and Asparagus Pasta	Ingredients: Salmon fillets, asparagus, whole wheat pasta, garlic, lemon zest, parsley, olive oil.
	Instructions: Cook pasta, sauté salmon and asparagus with garlic, lemon zest, and oil, toss with pasta and parsley.
	Preparation time: 30 minutes.
Turkey and Vegetable Chili	Ingredients: Ground turkey, kidney beans, tomatoes, bell peppers, onion, chili powder, cumin.
	Instructions: Brown turkey, add vegetables, beans, and spices, simmer until flavors meld.
	Preparation time: 45 minutes.
Mushroom and Spinach Stuffed Chicken	Ingredients: Chicken breasts, mushrooms, spinach, garlic, Parmesan cheese.

	Instructions: Sauté mushrooms and spinach with garlic and cheese, stuff into chicken, bake until cooked through.
	Preparation time: 35 minutes.
Lentil and Vegetable Curry	Ingredients: Lentils, carrots, cauliflower, onion, garlic, curry powder, vegetable broth, coconut milk
	Instructions: Simmer lentils and vegetables with curry powder, broth, and coconut milk until tender.
	Preparation time: 45 minutes.
Baked Cod with Tomato and Olive Relish	Ingredients: Cod fillets, tomatoes, olives, garlic, olive oil, parsley.
	Instructions: Mix tomatoes, olives, garlic, and oil, spoon over cod, bake until fish is flaky.
	Preparation time: 25 minutes.

Physical Exercises for Wellness

Exercise is essential for controlling ulcerative colitis (UC) because it improves general health, reduces symptoms, and improves quality of life. The main goal of this chapter is to provide a range of physical activities that are specifically designed to meet the special requirements and physical constraints of people with UC.

Recognizing the Advantages of Exercise: People with UC may benefit greatly from regular physical exercise in a number of ways, such as:

- Enhancing cardiovascular health: Exercise lowers the risk of heart disease and improves circulation by strengthening the heart and cardiovascular system.
- Improving mood and mental health: Exercise lowers stress and anxiety and releases endorphins, a class of neurotransmitters that encourage emotions of happiness and well-being.
- Weight management: By increasing metabolism, burning calories, and developing

muscular mass, exercise helps people control their weight.

- Supporting gastrointestinal health: Constipation and bloating symptoms may be reduced and bowel regularity can be encouraged with moderate activity.

- Strengthening bones and muscles: Weight-bearing activities and resistance training help preserve bone density, joint flexibility, and muscular strength, which lowers the risk of osteoporosis and frailty.

Guidelines for Safe and Efficient Exercise: It's crucial to put safety first and pay attention to your body while exercising if you have UC. Take into account these recommendations:

- Get started slowly: Start with low-impact workouts and increase frequency, length, and intensity gradually as your body tolerates it. Pay attention to your body's cues and modify your exercise regimen appropriately.

- Drink plenty of water: To avoid being dehydrated before and after exercise, particularly if you suffer from excessive fluid loss as a result of UC symptoms, make sure you consume enough of fluids.

- Pick enjoyable things to do: Choose pursuits that you find inspiring and enjoyable. Including your favorite activities dancing, yoga, swimming, or walking will boost your commitment and pleasure.

- Be mindful of your body: Pay attention to how your body feels after working out. If you feel pain, discomfort, or an aggravation of your UC symptoms, adjust or stop the exercise and see your doctor.

- Include diversity: To target various muscle groups, avoid boredom, and enhance general fitness and well-being, include a range of exercises in your regimen.

Physical Activities for UC Patients: The following physical activities are appropriate for people with UC:

1. Walking: To enhance cardiovascular health, elevate mood, and raise energy, go for quick walks outside or on a treadmill.

2. Swimming: For a low-impact, full-body exercise that tones muscles and improves cardiovascular fitness, swim laps or take part in water aerobics.

3. Yoga: To improve flexibility, lower stress levels, and encourage relaxation, practice mild yoga positions and breathing techniques.

4. Cycling: To increase endurance, cardiovascular fitness, and leg strength, ride a stationary bike or go on leisurely bike rides.

5. Tai Chi: Practice this peaceful martial art to reduce stress and promote relaxation while enhancing balance, flexibility, and mental concentration.

6. Pilates: To strengthen your core, correct posture, and increase your general body awareness, take Pilates courses or work on your own with mat exercises.

7. Resistance training: Perform strength training movements like squats, lunges, bicep curls,

and shoulder presses that target key muscle areas using resistance bands or small weights.

8. Stretching: Include stretches to increase range of motion, lessen tense muscles, and guard against injuries.

Recall that consistency is essential. Aim for 75 minutes of vigorous-intensity exercise or at least 150 minutes of moderate-intensity aerobic activity each week, in addition to two or more days of muscle-strengthening activities. Take note of your body's needs, drink enough of water, and enjoy the advantages of physical and mental well-being that come with exercise.

You may attain increased energy, resilience, and well-being with perseverance, patience, and self-care, enabling you to live your best life despite the difficulties posed by ulcerative colitis.

Conclusion

Individuals with ulcerative colitis (UC), which is characterized by persistent inflammation and ulcers in the colon and rectum, face a complicated terrain. UC management requires close attention to a number of variables, including as food choices, lifestyle modifications, and medicinal therapies. We explore the many facets of UC in this book with the goal of equipping readers with the information and tools they need to manage their illness well.

Comprehending the complex characteristics of UC is essential for formulating efficacious management strategies. Although the precise cause of the illness is still unknown, it is acknowledged as a chronic inflammatory bowel disease. Its development and course are thought to be influenced by a number of factors, including immunological dysregulation, environmental triggers, genetic predisposition, and changes in the gut flora. People may better customize management tactics to meet their requirements and get insight into the dynamics of their state by understanding these underlying processes.

Dietary concerns are crucial to the therapy of ulcerative colitis. The foods we eat have a significant impact on both our general health and symptoms of ulcerative colitis. Although there isn't a single diet that works for everyone with UC, following specific dietary guidelines may aid with inflammation reduction, symptom relief, and gut health promotion. A UC-friendly diet consists mostly of reducing possible triggers such processed meals, high-fat products, and specific carbs and emphasizing nutrient-dense foods like fruits, vegetables, lean meats, and healthy fats.

Developing a nutritious food plan specific to UC requires careful consideration of many different aspects. It includes choosing meals that are easy on the digestive tract, getting the most out of your nutritional intake, and avoiding situations that might make your symptoms worse. Timing meals, watching portion sizes, and staying hydrated are all important for supporting both symptom management and general health.

To help people put these dietary guidelines into practice, we provide a selection of breakfast dishes that are UC-compliant. These dishes are meant to be tasty, simple to make, and easy on the stomach. People may support their health journey with UC by starting their day on a good note by using healthy products and mindful cooking practices.

In summary, treating ulcerative colitis is a complex process that calls for an all-encompassing strategy. People with ulcerative colitis (UC) may improve their overall quality of life, improve symptom management, and encourage healing by learning about the complexity of the condition, adopting good lifestyle practices, and making educated food decisions. People may overcome the difficulties presented by UC and flourish in spite of its effects if they are committed, resilient, and get continuous support from family and friends.